The Urban Gardener's Handbook

Growing Your Own Food in the City

Jonas Mayer

Copyright Information

Table of Contents

Introduction

In the bustling, crowded cities of today, where concrete jungles stretch as far as the eye can see, the idea of growing one's own food might seem ambitious, if not impossible. Yet, urban gardening is an increasingly popular and practical solution for people looking to cultivate their own food amidst limited space. Not only does it offer fresh and nutritious produce, but it also fosters a sense of community, sustainability, and connection to nature.

This essay explores the reasons behind

the growing trend of urban gardening, the myriad benefits it brings to city dwellers, and the challenges one might face while taking up this rewarding endeavor.

Why Grow Your Own Food in the City?

Urban living often disconnects people from the natural world. Store-bought produce is usually grown far away, transported over long distances, and subject to processing and preservation techniques. As a result, the food we consume often lacks the freshness and nutrient density of homegrown options. By growing their own food, city residents can regain control over what they eat, ensuring quality, freshness, and even organic standards.

Furthermore, growing food in urban areas addresses critical issues like food security and environmental sustainability. City populations are rapidly increasing, leading to growing demand for resources, particularly food. Urban gardening can help reduce dependence on industrial agriculture by making food production hyper-local. It reduces the carbon footprint associated with transportation and packaging while also mitigating urban heat islands through greenery.

Urban gardening is also empowering. It transforms balconies, rooftops, and small patches of land into thriving ecosystems where food can be cultivated. The ability to grow one's own food, even in small quantities, fosters a sense of independence and accomplishment.

The Benefits of Urban Gardening

1. Access to Fresh, Healthy Food

Urban gardening provides direct access to fresh, organic, and chemical-free produce.

Homegrown fruits, vegetables, and herbs retain their full nutritional value because they are consumed shortly after harvesting. This freshness contrasts sharply with store-bought produce, which can sit in transport and storage for days or even weeks before reaching consumers.

Additionally, growing your own food encourages healthier eating habits. When you have access to a variety of fresh greens, vegetables, and herbs, you're more likely to incorporate them into your meals. The act of gardening itself also fosters mindfulness about diet and nutrition.

2. Cost-Effectiveness

While the initial setup for an urban garden may involve some investment in tools, soil, and seeds, the long-term financial benefits are significant. Urban gardening can help reduce grocery bills, especially for expensive organic produce. For instance, a small herb garden can yield a constant supply of basil, mint, or parsley, which are often pricey at supermarkets. Similarly, cultivating vegetables like tomatoes, lettuce, and peppers can save money over time.

3. Environmental Benefits

Urban gardening contributes to environmental conservation in multiple ways. By growing food locally, city dwellers reduce their reliance on industrial farming, which is resource-intensive and contributes significantly to greenhouse gas emissions. Gardening also promotes composting, turning organic kitchen waste into nutrient-rich soil instead of adding to landfill waste.

Moreover, urban gardens serve as green spaces that improve air quality and reduce urban heat. Plants absorb carbon dioxide and release oxygen, making cities healthier and more livable. They also help manage rainwater by reducing runoff, preventing flooding in heavily paved areas.

4. Improved Mental and Physical Health

Gardening is a form of exercise that promotes physical well-being. Activities like digging, planting, and watering provide moderate physical activity, which is especially valuable in urban settings where access to green outdoor spaces can be limited.

The mental health benefits of gardening are equally profound. Spending time with plants reduces stress, anxiety, and depression. The act of nurturing a plant and watching it grow fosters a sense of accomplishment and joy. Urban gardens also provide an escape from the noise and pace of city life, offering a tranquil space to unwind and reconnect with nature.

5. Building Community Connections

Urban gardening often brings people together, especially in shared spaces like community gardens or rooftop plots. These spaces encourage collaboration, knowledge-sharing, and a sense of community. Neighbors can share resources, gardening tips, and even harvests, fostering stronger social bonds.

In addition, urban gardening can have a positive social impact. It can be an educational tool for teaching children about food systems, sustainability, and the importance of healthy eating. It can also be a platform for addressing issues like food deserts in underprivileged areas, providing access to fresh produce where grocery stores are scarce.

Challenges and How to Overcome Them

While urban gardening offers immense benefits, it is not without its challenges. Limited space, access to resources, and environmental factors can make growing food in cities a daunting task. However, these obstacles can be overcome with creativity, knowledge, and determination.

1. Limited Space

Space is often the biggest challenge for urban gardeners. Apartments with no balconies or small backyards may seem ill-suited for gardening. However, innovative techniques like vertical gardening, container gardening, and rooftop gardening can maximize available space. Vertical gardens use trellises, shelves, and hanging pots to grow plants upward, making them ideal for small spaces. Container gardening allows plants to thrive in pots or grow bags, which can be easily moved to optimize sunlight exposure.

2. Lack of Sunlight

Many urban spaces are shaded by tall buildings, limiting sunlight—a critical factor for plant growth. Selecting shade-tolerant plants like lettuce, spinach, and herbs can help address this issue. For indoor gardening, investing in grow lights can ensure plants receive adequate light.

3. Soil Quality

Urban soil is often contaminated with pollutants, making it unsuitable for growing food. Container gardening offers a solution by allowing gardeners to use clean, store-bought soil mixes. Raised garden beds with fresh soil can also create safe, fertile environments for plants.

4. Water Management

Access to water and efficient irrigation can be challenging in cities. Urban gardeners can practice water conservation techniques like mulching to retain soil moisture and installing drip irrigation systems for precise watering. Collecting rainwater in barrels is another eco-friendly solution.

5. Pests and Diseases

Urban gardens are not immune to pests and diseases, especially in densely populated areas. Using natural pest control methods like neem oil, companion planting, and introducing beneficial insects (e.g., ladybugs) can keep infestations under control. Regular monitoring and prompt action can also minimize damage.

6. Time Constraints

Many urban dwellers lead busy lives, making it difficult to dedicate time to gardening. However, low-maintenance plants and automated systems like self-watering pots can help reduce the effort required. Even spending just a few minutes a day tending to plants can make a difference.

Urban gardening is a transformative practice that empowers city dwellers to grow their own food while reaping environmental, health, and social benefits. Despite challenges like limited space and resources, innovative solutions and determination make it possible for anyone to succeed. By turning unused spaces into productive gardens, urban residents can contribute to a greener, healthier, and more self-reliant future.

Whether you're growing herbs on a windowsill or cultivating a rooftop oasis, urban gardening is a journey worth embarking on—for yourself, your community, and the planet.

Part 1

Getting Started

Urban gardening offers a creative and sustainable way to grow your own food in the limited spaces available in cities. It allows city dwellers to reconnect with nature, produce fresh and healthy food, and contribute to environmental sustainability. Whether you are a beginner or an experienced gardener, understanding the essentials of urban gardening, planning your space effectively, and choosing the right tools are key steps to success. This essay explores the core principles of urban gardening, including what it is, the different gardening styles, how to plan your garden, and the tools and materials needed for urban gardening.

Understanding Urban Gardening

What Is Urban Gardening?

Urban gardening refers to the practice of growing plants—ranging from vegetables and herbs to flowers and fruits—within urban environments. This form of gardening utilizes available spaces in cities, such as balconies, rooftops, windowsills, and even vacant lots, to cultivate food and greenery. Urban gardening has become increasingly popular due to the rise in food sustainability awareness and a desire to live healthier, more self-sufficient lifestyles in cities.

Urban gardening allows individuals to grow their own food, reducing reliance on industrial farming, transportation, and commercial agriculture. It contributes to the reduction of food miles, minimizes packaging waste, and provides fresh, organic produce. Additionally, urban gardening encourages a sense of community by transforming urban spaces into green areas that promote mental well-being and environmental consciousness.

Different Styles: Balcony, Rooftop, Vertical, and Indoor Gardening

Urban gardening comes in many styles, each suited to different living conditions and spaces. Understanding the different methods allows you to choose the right one based on your specific needs.

1. Balcony Gardening

Balcony gardening is one of the most accessible styles of urban gardening. A balcony provides an elevated space that receives plenty of sunlight, making it ideal for growing plants. From small herb pots to larger container gardens, balconies can accommodate a wide range of plants. The key to balcony gardening is choosing the right containers and ensuring proper drainage to prevent waterlogging.

2. Rooftop Gardening

Rooftop gardening takes advantage of unused space atop buildings. It provides ample sunlight, often unrestricted by surrounding buildings. Rooftop gardens can support a wide range of crops, from leafy greens and herbs to small fruit trees. However, rooftop gardening requires considerations for safety, structural integrity, and potential wind exposure. Containers, raised beds, and hydroponic systems are common solutions used for rooftop gardening.

3. Vertical Gardening

Vertical gardening is a space-saving technique that maximizes vertical surfaces to grow plants. Using walls, trellises, fences, or vertical planters, gardeners can grow plants upwards instead of outwards. This method is ideal for small spaces like apartments, where horizontal space is limited. Plants such as tomatoes, cucumbers, and climbing beans thrive in vertical gardens. Additionally, vertical gardening allows for efficient use of sunlight and can increase plant yield in confined spaces.

4. Indoor Gardening

Indoor gardening is perfect for those with limited outdoor space or living in apartments with minimal access to natural light. Growing plants indoors can be done with the help of containers, window boxes, and grow lights. Indoor gardeners often focus on herbs, microgreens, or small vegetables that do not require a lot of space. Hydroponics and aquaponics are also effective indoor gardening methods, as they do not require soil, making them ideal for limited spaces.

Each of these gardening styles has its benefits and can be adapted to the unique needs of the urban gardener. Choosing the right style depends on the available space, light conditions, and the type of plants you wish to grow.

Planning Your Urban Garden

Assessing Space, Light, and Water Availability

Before you start planting, it is essential to assess the space you have available. Urban environments often offer limited space, so understanding how to make the most of your area is crucial to your garden's success.

1. Space

Urban gardening often takes place in small areas like balconies, windowsills, rooftops, or shared community spaces. To begin planning, assess the available space for gardening. Consider whether your area can accommodate raised beds, containers, or vertical structures. Measure the space to estimate how many plants you can realistically grow and plan accordingly.

2. Light

Light is one of the most important factors when planning an urban garden. Most plants need at least 6-8 hours of direct sunlight per day to grow successfully. Evaluate the light exposure in your space by observing where the sun hits during the day. Balconies and rooftops typically receive more direct sunlight, while shaded areas or spaces with limited access to sunlight may require supplementary lighting, such as grow lights. Indoor gardening also requires the careful selection of plants that thrive in low-light conditions or the use of artificial lighting to supplement natural light.

3. Water Availability

Watering is crucial for the success of any garden. Assessing your water supply is essential to ensure that your plants get enough moisture. In urban environments, water may not always be readily available. Ensure that you have easy access to water, whether it's through a hose, watering can, or rainwater harvesting system. Urban gardens, especially rooftop gardens, may benefit from rainwater collection systems to minimize water usage and reduce utility costs. Be mindful of the specific water needs of the plants you're growing and plan an irrigation system accordingly.

Choosing the Right Location
Choosing the right location for your urban garden involves more than just light and space. You should consider factors like temperature, wind exposure, and the potential for pests.

Temperature: Urban areas tend to have a higher ambient temperature than rural areas, which is known as the urban heat island effect. This can be both an advantage and a disadvantage, depending on the type of plants you want to grow. It is essential to select plants that can tolerate higher temperatures, especially if you're growing on a rooftop or exposed balcony.

Wind: Rooftop gardens or high-altitude balconies may experience strong winds, which can stress plants. If wind is a concern, consider using windbreaks, tall planters, or trellises to protect your plants from gusts.

Pests and Pollution: Urban areas may have higher levels of air pollution and pests, which can affect plant health. Consider using natural pest control methods like neem oil or companion planting to mitigate pest problems. Avoid growing plants that are highly sensitive to pollutants if you live in a highly polluted area.

Designing for Aesthetic and Productivity

Designing your urban garden should strike a balance between aesthetics and productivity. Urban gardens don't just need to be functional—they should also be pleasant spaces to relax and enjoy. Begin by considering the style and layout of your garden.

Aesthetic Considerations: Think about how your garden will enhance your outdoor space. Incorporate a variety of plants, including flowering herbs, colorful vegetables, and decorative elements like garden statues or fairy lights. Vertical gardening can add an artistic touch by allowing you to grow plants on walls or fences.

Maximizing Productivity: Focus on creating an efficient garden layout that maximizes your space's potential. Companion planting, which involves pairing plants that support each other's growth, can boost productivity and reduce the need for pesticides. Plan your garden so that taller plants are placed at the back, while shorter plants or herbs occupy the front row. Raised beds and container gardening are great options for ensuring productivity in smaller spaces.

Essential Tools and Materials

Basic Gardening Tools for Urban Spaces

While urban gardening does not require a vast array of tools, there are some essentials that will make your gardening experience much easier. A few key tools include:

1. Hand Trowel: Perfect for digging, planting, and moving soil.

2. Pruners: For trimming and maintaining healthy plants.

3. Watering Can or Hose: Ensure proper watering without waste.

4. Gloves: Protect your hands from thorns, dirt, and potential irritants.

5. Soil and Compost: High-quality soil and compost are crucial for healthy plant growth.

Containers, Raised Beds, and Vertical Structures

Urban gardening often requires the use of containers, raised beds, or vertical structures to make the most of limited space.

1. Containers: These come in various sizes

and materials, including plastic, ceramic, and terracotta. Choose containers with good drainage to prevent waterlogging. Containers are perfect for growing herbs, vegetables, and even small fruit-bearing plants.

2. Raised Beds: Raised beds are ideal for urban gardens where the soil quality is poor or where you want to create a more structured garden. They provide better drainage and allow for the easy customization of soil and compost.

3. Vertical Structures: Use trellises, vertical planters, or repurposed materials

like pallets to grow plants upwards. Vertical gardening maximizes space and can be aesthetically pleasing, adding an element of creativity to your garden.

Budget-Friendly Tips

Urban gardening doesn't need to be expensive. There are several ways to create a thriving garden on a budget:

DIY Containers: Repurpose old containers, like plastic bottles, wooden crates, or even old shoe racks, for growing plants.

Composting: Start composting food scraps

and yard waste to create nutrient-rich soil for your plants.

Rainwater Harvesting: Set up a simple rainwater collection system to water your garden and reduce your water bill.

Starting an urban garden requires careful planning, the right tools, and a little creativity. By understanding urban gardening styles, assessing your space and light availability, and selecting the appropriate tools and materials, you can turn even the smallest urban space into a thriving garden. Whether you choose balcony, rooftop, vertical, or indoor gardening, the possibilities are endless. Embrace the challenge and start your urban gardening journey today.

Part 2

Growing Your Food

Urban gardening requires thoughtful planning and execution to maximize limited spaces and resources. Growing your own food, whether vegetables, fruits, herbs, or edible flowers, is a rewarding journey that demands knowledge about plant selection, soil health, water management, and pest control. This section provides a comprehensive guide to choosing the right crops, preparing the soil, managing water efficiently, and addressing common challenges like pests and diseases.

Choosing What to Grow

Vegetables, Herbs, Fruits, and Edible Flowers

When deciding what to grow in your urban garden, the key is to choose plants that align with your space, climate, and personal preferences. Urban gardening is highly versatile, and even small spaces can yield an impressive variety of crops.

Vegetables:

Growing vegetables is a popular choice for urban gardeners. Leafy greens like spinach, kale, and lettuce thrive in containers and grow quickly. Tomatoes, peppers, and cucumbers are excellent options for slightly larger spaces or vertical gardens. Root vegetables such as radishes and carrots can also be grown in deep pots.

Herbs:
Herbs like basil, mint, parsley, and thyme are ideal for small urban spaces due to their compact size and versatility in cooking. They grow well in containers, require minimal maintenance, and can

thrive on windowsills or balconies.

Fruits:

Urban gardeners with more space, such as a rooftop or large balcony, can grow fruits like strawberries, dwarf citrus trees, and blueberries. Compact fruit varieties are often designed specifically for container gardening.

Edible Flowers:

Edible flowers like nasturtiums, violets, and calendula add color and beauty to urban gardens while being functional in culinary applications. They grow easily in pots and can enhance the aesthetic appeal of your garden.

Climate and Seasonal Considerations

Understanding your local climate and growing seasons is essential for successful urban gardening. Each plant has specific temperature and light requirements that must be met for optimal growth.

Warm-Season Crops: Tomatoes, peppers, cucumbers, and melons thrive in warm temperatures and require plenty of sunlight.

Cool-Season Crops: Spinach, lettuce, and

broccoli prefer cooler temperatures and can be planted during spring or fall.

If your city has unpredictable weather, consider growing plants in portable containers that can be moved indoors during extreme conditions. Additionally, using greenhouses, cold frames, or grow lights can extend your growing season and protect sensitive crops.

Companion Planting for Small Spaces

Companion planting is a technique that involves growing compatible plants together to maximize space, improve plant health, and deter pests. It is particularly useful for urban gardens with limited space.

Examples of Companion Plants:

Tomatoes and Basil: Basil repels pests and enhances the flavor of tomatoes.

Carrots and Onions: Onions deter carrot flies.

Marigolds and Vegetables: Marigolds repel nematodes and aphids.

Companion planting also helps in

managing soil nutrients effectively, as certain plants replenish nutrients that others consume.

Soil, Compost, and Fertilizers

Building Healthy Soil in the City

Healthy soil is the foundation of a thriving garden. Urban soil, however, often lacks nutrients or is contaminated by pollutants. For urban gardening, it's best to use clean, store-bought soil or create your own soil mix using compost and organic matter.

Soil Mix for Containers: A good mix includes equal parts of potting soil, compost, and perlite or sand for drainage. Adding coco coir helps retain moisture.

Testing Soil Quality: Use a soil test kit to check pH levels and nutrient content, ensuring it's suitable for your chosen plants.

Composting in Small Spaces

Composting is an eco-friendly way to recycle kitchen and garden waste into nutrient-rich soil. Even in small urban spaces, composting is achievable with the right techniques.

Options for Small-Space Composting:

Vermicomposting: Using worms to break down organic waste. Worm bins are compact and odor-free, making them ideal for apartments.

Bokashi Composting: This method ferments organic waste in airtight containers, requiring minimal space.

Compost Tumbler: A small, enclosed compost bin that accelerates decomposition.

Adding compost to your soil improves its structure, fertility, and ability to retain moisture, creating an optimal environment for plant growth.

Organic Fertilizers and Natural Soil Amendments

Chemical fertilizers are often unnecessary in urban gardening. Organic fertilizers and natural amendments provide essential nutrients without harming the environment.

Popular Organic Fertilizers:

Compost Tea: A nutrient-rich liquid made from steeping compost in water.

Bone Meal: A source of phosphorus for root development.

Seaweed Extract: Provides trace minerals and boosts plant health.

Amendments like eggshells (for calcium) and coffee grounds (for nitrogen) can be added directly to soil, enhancing its nutrient profile.

Watering and Irrigation

Efficient Watering Techniques

Watering is a critical aspect of urban gardening, especially in small containers that dry out quickly. Proper techniques ensure that plants receive enough hydration without waste.

Watering Tips:

Water plants early in the morning or late in the evening to minimize evaporation.

Use a watering can or hose with a gentle spray nozzle to avoid disturbing the soil.

Mulch the soil surface to retain moisture and reduce watering frequency.

DIY Drip Irrigation for Urban Gardens

Drip irrigation is an efficient method of delivering water directly to plant roots, reducing waste and ensuring consistent hydration. Creating a DIY drip irrigation system is simple and cost-effective.

How to Make a DIY Drip System:

Use recycled plastic bottles or buckets to create a reservoir.

Attach tubing with small holes near the plant roots to control water flow.

Position the system to deliver water slowly over time.

Saving Water in Urban Environments

Urban gardeners can adopt water-saving practices to reduce their environmental impact:

Collect rainwater in barrels or buckets

for irrigation.

Use self-watering containers with reservoirs to minimize water loss.

Group plants with similar water needs together to simplify watering.

Pest and Disease Management

Urban gardens are not immune to pests and diseases, which can damage crops if not addressed promptly. Fortunately, there are natural and organic methods to manage these issues effectively.

Common Urban Gardening Pests and How to Manage Them

Some of the most common pests encountered in urban gardens include:

Aphids: Small insects that suck plant sap. Manage them by spraying plants with a mix of water and mild soap.

Spider Mites: Tiny pests that cause yellowing leaves. Neem oil is an effective remedy.

Slugs and Snails: These can be deterred by placing crushed eggshells or copper tape around plants.

Natural and Organic Remedies

Avoid chemical pesticides in urban gardens to protect your health and the environment. Instead, use:

Neem Oil: A natural pesticide that controls a variety of pests.

Garlic Spray: Deters pests with its strong smell.

Diatomaceous Earth: A powder that damages pests' exoskeletons, effectively killing them.

Introduce beneficial insects like ladybugs and lacewings, which prey on harmful pests, to create a balanced ecosystem in your garden.

Preventive Measures for a Healthy Garden

Prevention is the best approach to managing pests and diseases.

Keep plants healthy by providing adequate sunlight, water, and nutrients.

Remove weeds and debris, which can

harbor pests.

Rotate crops each season to prevent the buildup of soil-borne diseases.

Growing your own food in an urban setting requires careful planning and consistent effort, but the rewards are immense. By selecting the right crops, building healthy soil, managing water wisely, and addressing pests and diseases naturally, urban gardeners can create thriving and sustainable gardens. This section equips you with the knowledge to turn any small space into a productive green haven, contributing to your health, environment, and community.

Part 3

Advanced Techniques

Urban gardening often involves creative solutions to maximize space and resources. Advanced techniques like vertical gardening, rooftop and balcony setups, and indoor gardening are particularly suited to urban environments. They allow gardeners to grow more food in limited areas while maintaining sustainability and functionality. This section explores these innovative methods, guiding you on how to transform even the smallest spaces into lush and productive gardens.

Vertical Gardening

Vertical gardening is a transformative technique that utilizes vertical space to grow plants. This method is perfect for urban gardeners with limited horizontal space, such as balconies, small yards, or even bare walls.

Creative Ideas for Growing Upward

Vertical gardening is not only practical but also visually appealing. Here are some creative ideas to help you get started:

Wall-Mounted Planters: Attach pots or pockets to walls or fences for growing herbs, flowers, or small vegetables like lettuce.

Trellises and Arbors: Use trellises to support climbing plants like tomatoes, peas, or cucumbers. Arbors are ideal for gourds or flowering vines.

Hanging Baskets: Hang baskets filled with cascading plants such as strawberries, cherry tomatoes, or herbs like mint.

Pallet Gardens: Recycle old wooden pallets by attaching small pots or filling the gaps with soil to create a unique vertical garden.

Tower Gardens: Stack pots or containers to create garden towers. These are especially effective for growing root vegetables like radishes or onions.

Best Plants for Vertical Gardens

Not all plants are suitable for vertical gardening. The best choices are those that are lightweight, compact, or naturally vining.

Climbing Plants: Beans, peas, and

cucumbers grow vertically with support.

Trailing Plants: Strawberries, sweet potatoes, and nasturtiums work well in hanging baskets.

Compact Crops: Herbs like basil, thyme, and parsley thrive in small containers.

Flowers: Edible flowers such as pansies or marigolds add beauty and functionality.

DIY Vertical Planters

Building your own vertical planters is an affordable and customizable option.

PVC Pipe Planters: Drill holes in large PVC pipes and fill them with soil to grow herbs or lettuce.

Bottle Planters: Cut and stack plastic bottles to create a tiered system for small plants.

Wooden Frames: Build a frame with shelves or grids to hold pots securely.

With vertical gardening, the possibilities are endless. This method not only maximizes space but also enhances urban aesthetics.

Rooftop and Balcony Gardening

Rooftop and balcony gardening offer urban gardeners the opportunity to utilize underused spaces for food production. These setups require thoughtful planning to ensure safety, efficiency, and sustainability.

Setting Up a Rooftop Garden: Safety and Structural Considerations

Rooftop gardening requires a careful assessment of your roof's structural integrity and load-bearing capacity.

Safety First: Consult a structural engineer to determine if your roof can handle the weight of soil, water, and plants. Lightweight containers and soil mixes can reduce strain.

Waterproofing: Protect your roof from water damage by installing a waterproof barrier or membrane beneath the garden setup.

Wind Protection: Rooftops are often windy, which can damage plants. Use windbreaks like trellises, mesh screens, or strategically placed plants to shield sensitive crops.

Once these considerations are addressed, create a layout that includes pathways, drainage systems, and designated planting areas.

Maximizing Small Balconies for Food Production

Balconies, no matter how small, can become productive gardens with strategic planning.

Container Gardening: Use pots, tubs, or grow bags for versatile planting options. Select lightweight materials to prevent overloading the balcony.

Shelving Units: Install shelves to stack containers vertically, optimizing space while keeping plants accessible.

Hanging Planters: Suspend planters from railings or ceiling hooks to create additional growing space.

Multifunctional Furniture: Use furniture with built-in planters or storage for gardening supplies to save space.

By integrating vertical gardening techniques, balcony gardens can accommodate a surprising variety of crops, including leafy greens, herbs, and even dwarf fruit trees.

Indoor Gardening

Indoor gardening is an ideal solution for urban dwellers with limited outdoor access. With the right tools and techniques, you can grow a wide variety of plants inside your home, transforming it into a green oasis.

Growing with Limited Light: LED and Grow Lights

One of the biggest challenges of indoor

gardening is the lack of natural sunlight. Grow lights, particularly LED lights, provide a solution by mimicking the light spectrum needed for photosynthesis.

Types of Grow Lights:

LED Lights: Energy-efficient, long-lasting, and customizable to specific wavelengths.

Fluorescent Lights: Affordable and effective for small-scale indoor gardens.

High-Intensity Discharge (HID) Lights: Suitable for larger setups but consume more energy.

Placement and Timing: Position lights 6-12 inches above plants and keep them on for 12-16 hours a day, depending on the plant's needs. Use timers for consistent lighting schedules.

Herbs and Microgreens for Indoor Spaces

Herbs and microgreens are perfect for indoor gardening due to their compact size and quick growth.

Popular Herbs: Basil, cilantro, parsley, and chives grow well in small pots on windowsills or shelves.

Microgreens: These nutrient-dense greens, like arugula, radish, and sunflower shoots, can be grown in shallow trays with minimal soil.

Indoor herb gardens not only provide fresh ingredients but also improve air quality and add greenery to your living space.

Hydroponics and Aquaponics

For a high-tech approach to indoor gardening, hydroponics and aquaponics offer efficient ways to grow plants without soil.

Hydroponics:

Plants are grown in a nutrient-rich water solution.

Systems like deep water culture (DWC), nutrient film technique (NFT), and aeroponics cater to different scales and needs.

Ideal for crops like lettuce, spinach, and strawberries.

Aquaponics:

Combines hydroponics with aquaculture,

using fish to provide natural nutrients for plants.

The system creates a symbiotic relationship between plants and fish, making it highly sustainable.

These methods are space-efficient, environmentally friendly, and capable of producing high yields year-round. While the initial setup costs may be higher, the long-term benefits make them a worthwhile investment for dedicated urban gardeners.

Advanced gardening techniques like vertical gardening, rooftop and balcony setups, and indoor systems expand the possibilities for urban food production. These methods demonstrate that limited space is no obstacle to creating a thriving, sustainable garden. By thinking creatively and leveraging modern tools and practices, urban dwellers can grow fresh, healthy food while contributing to a greener cityscape.

Part 4

Harvesting and Beyond

The journey of urban gardening does not end with planting and nurturing crops. Harvesting, storing, and extending the use of your produce are vital steps that ensure the fruits of your labor are fully enjoyed. Additionally, incorporating sustainable practices into urban gardening has a profound impact, not only on your household but also on the community and environment. This section explores effective methods for harvesting, preserving, and promoting sustainability in urban gardening.

Harvesting and Storing Your Produce

A successful urban gardening journey culminates in the harvest. Knowing the right time and methods to pick your produce is crucial for flavor, nutrition, and yield. Equally important is how you store and preserve it to minimize waste.

Knowing When to Harvest

Each crop has its own indicators of ripeness, which vary depending on the plant type and intended use. Here are general guidelines for harvesting:

Leafy Greens: Harvest when leaves are large enough to eat but before they become bitter or start bolting. For crops like spinach, kale, and lettuce, use the "cut-and-come-again" method by snipping outer leaves while leaving the inner ones to grow.

Root Vegetables: Check size by gently feeling the top of the root just above the soil. Carrots, radishes, and beets should be firm and brightly colored when harvested.

Fruits and Tomatoes: Pick fruits like strawberries, tomatoes, or cucumbers when they are fully colored and fragrant. For green vegetables like zucchini, harvest when they are still small for the best taste.

Herbs: Harvest herbs like basil, mint, and parsley early in the morning for maximum flavor. Snip stems just above a set of leaves to encourage regrowth.

Edible Flowers: Collect flowers such as nasturtiums or marigolds when they are freshly bloomed for peak flavor and aesthetics.

Delaying harvest can lead to overripe or tough produce, so it's important to observe your garden daily and make timely picks.

Tips for Storing Fresh Produce

Proper storage helps maintain the quality and lifespan of your harvest. Follow these tips to keep your produce fresh:

Refrigeration: Store leafy greens, root vegetables, and herbs in the refrigerator. Wrap them in a damp paper towel to prevent wilting.

Cool, Dark Places: Potatoes, onions, and

garlic should be kept in a cool, dark, and dry space. Avoid storing them together, as certain vegetables release ethylene gas, which can cause spoilage.

Use Airtight Containers: Store fruits like berries in airtight containers lined with paper towels to absorb excess moisture.

Short-Term Storage: Eat delicate produce like berries and greens within a few days to enjoy their full flavor and nutrition.

Preserving: Freezing, Drying, and Canning

Preservation techniques allow you to

extend the shelf life of your harvest while maintaining flavor and nutrition. Here are three popular methods:

Freezing:

Ideal for leafy greens, fruits, and herbs. Blanch vegetables briefly in boiling water before freezing to retain color and texture.

Freeze herbs in ice cube trays with water or olive oil for quick use in soups and stews.

Drying:

Use a dehydrator or oven to dry herbs, tomatoes, or fruits. Store them in airtight containers to protect from moisture.

Sun-drying is another sustainable option, though it requires consistent sunlight.

Canning:

Preserve jams, pickles, and sauces using sterilized jars and boiling water baths. Follow safety guidelines to prevent contamination.

Pressure canning is recommended for low-acid vegetables like beans or carrots.

These preservation methods are essential for urban gardeners aiming to enjoy their harvest year-round.

Sustainability in Urban Gardening

Sustainability is at the heart of urban gardening. By reducing waste, recycling resources, and fostering community connections, gardeners can make a meaningful contribution to the environment and society.

Reducing Waste and Recycling in the Garden

Urban gardening provides ample opportunities to practice waste reduction:

Composting:

Turn kitchen scraps, garden clippings, and coffee grounds into nutrient-rich compost. Small-scale compost bins or worm farms are perfect for urban spaces.

Reusing Containers:

Use old pots, buckets, or even repurposed

household items like jars and cans as plant containers.

Rainwater Harvesting:

Collect rainwater in barrels or containers for irrigation, reducing reliance on municipal water supplies.

Repurposing Waste:

Use crushed eggshells as a natural fertilizer or pest deterrent. Banana peels can also enrich the soil with potassium.

By adopting these practices, urban gardeners can minimize their ecological footprint while improving their garden's productivity.

Community Gardening: Sharing Resources and Knowledge

Community gardens are vibrant spaces where urban gardeners come together to share resources, knowledge, and experiences. These initiatives foster collaboration and sustainability:

Shared Resources:

Community gardens often provide shared tools, composting facilities, and water sources, reducing costs for individual gardeners.

Skill Exchange:

Experienced gardeners can mentor beginners, sharing tips on planting, pest control, and sustainable practices.

Group Activities:

Workshops, seed exchanges, and communal harvest celebrations bring people together, strengthening community bonds.

Community gardening is not only about growing food but also about nurturing relationships and creating green spaces in urban areas.

Long-Term Benefits for Your Community and the Environment

Urban gardening has far-reaching benefits beyond personal food production. Here are some long-term impacts:

Environmental Impact:

Urban gardens reduce the heat island effect by adding greenery to cities, improving air quality and reducing energy consumption for cooling.

They also promote biodiversity by providing habitats for pollinators like bees and butterflies.

Food Security:

Growing food locally reduces reliance on industrial agriculture and long supply chains, ensuring fresher and healthier produce.

In food deserts, urban gardens provide access to affordable, nutritious food.

Social Equity:

Community gardening initiatives empower underserved communities by offering access to land, education, and fresh produce.

Mental Health and Well-Being:

Gardening reduces stress and promotes physical activity. Community gardens also provide safe spaces for social interaction and recreation.

Harvesting and preserving your produce is a rewarding culmination of the urban gardening process, while sustainability ensures that the practice has lasting positive effects. By mastering techniques like freezing and canning, reducing waste, and engaging in community gardening, urban gardeners contribute to a healthier, greener world. Through their efforts, they not only feed themselves but also inspire others to embrace the joys and responsibilities of cultivating their own food.

Conclusion

Urban gardening is more than a practical solution for growing food in limited spaces; it is a transformative journey that fosters self-reliance, creativity, and sustainability. Reflecting on your progress, envisioning the growth of your garden, and understanding its role in the future of urban food production can deepen your appreciation for this rewarding practice.

Reflecting on Your Gardening Journey

Every urban gardener's journey is unique, shaped by individual circumstances, creativity, and perseverance. Looking back on the process offers valuable insights into your progress and the skills you've gained.

Personal Growth and Skills

Starting an urban garden may have seemed daunting, but each challenge you overcame has contributed to your development. Perhaps you learned to optimize limited space, mastered composting, or nurtured your first crop of fresh tomatoes. Beyond practical skills, gardening teaches patience, problem-solving, and adaptability. Whether you created a lush balcony garden, a productive rooftop plot, or a cozy indoor herb corner, your garden is a reflection of your dedication and effort.

A Connection with Nature

Urban environments often feel detached from the natural world, but gardening bridges this gap. Watching plants grow, observing pollinators like bees, and feeling the soil in your hands instills a deeper connection to nature. This bond promotes mindfulness and helps reduce stress, making gardening a therapeutic experience.

Overcoming Challenges

Reflect on the obstacles you faced—whether it was pests, poor lighting, or limited space—and the creative solutions you implemented. Perhaps you built a vertical garden, set up a drip irrigation system, or experimented with organic pest control methods. Each challenge was an opportunity to grow as a gardener, leaving you better equipped for future endeavors.

The Joy of Harvest

One of the most fulfilling moments in urban gardening is harvesting your produce. The satisfaction of plucking fresh herbs or enjoying homegrown vegetables at your table validates your hard work. These experiences highlight the tangible rewards of gardening and remind us of the importance of self-sufficiency.

Reflecting on your gardening journey reveals how far you've come and sets the stage for even greater achievements.

Expanding Your Urban Garden

As your confidence and skills grow, you may want to expand your garden. Urban gardening offers endless possibilities for scaling up, diversifying, and enriching your setup.

Adding New Plants

Expanding your plant selection can increase your garden's productivity and variety. Consider introducing:

Perennials: Plants like asparagus,

strawberries, and herbs that yield produce year after year.

Exotic Crops: Experiment with unique plants like figs, ginger, or lemongrass that add diversity to your harvest.

Pollinator-Friendly Plants: Include flowers like lavender or sunflowers to attract bees and butterflies, enhancing biodiversity.

Exploring Advanced Techniques

Take your gardening to the next level with innovative practices:

Hydroponics and Aquaponics: These soil-free systems maximize space and yield, making them ideal for urban gardeners seeking efficiency.

Permaculture Design: Incorporate sustainable practices such as companion planting, water recycling, and natural pest control to create a self-sustaining garden ecosystem.

Vertical and Modular Gardening: Expand your vertical garden or invest in modular systems that allow you to rearrange and optimize your space.

Collaborating with the Community

Expanding your garden can also mean connecting with others:

Community Gardens: Join or start a community garden to share resources, learn from others, and grow collectively.

Workshops and Events: Organize or attend gardening workshops to exchange knowledge and inspire others to embrace urban gardening.

Sustainability Goals

As you expand, focus on sustainability by incorporating practices like composting, rainwater harvesting, and reducing plastic usage in your garden. These measures ensure that your garden contributes positively to the environment.

Growth in urban gardening is not just about size but also about creating a more diverse, efficient, and sustainable system.

The Future of Urban Food Production

Urban gardening is not just a personal endeavor; it is part of a broader movement to address global challenges related to food security, climate change, and urbanization. Its role in shaping the future of food production is significant and growing.

Addressing Food Insecurity

As urban populations rise, the demand for food increases, placing strain on traditional agriculture and supply chains. Urban gardening offers a localized solution by:

Increasing Access to Fresh Produce: Urban gardens provide healthy, affordable food in areas where fresh produce is scarce.

Reducing Dependence on Imports: By growing food locally, cities can reduce reliance on imported goods, stabilizing food systems during crises.

Combating Climate Change

Urban gardening helps mitigate climate change in several ways:

Carbon Sequestration: Plants absorb carbon dioxide, reducing the carbon footprint of urban areas.

Cooling Effect: Green spaces lower urban temperatures, reducing the need for energy-intensive cooling systems.

Waste Reduction: Composting organic waste reduces landfill contributions and methane emissions.

Promoting Sustainable Living

Urban gardening fosters sustainable practices that extend beyond the garden:

Reduced Food Miles: Growing food locally eliminates the energy and emissions associated with transportation and packaging.

Resource Efficiency: Techniques like drip irrigation and hydroponics maximize resource use while minimizing waste.

Community Engagement: Gardening initiatives promote environmental awareness and encourage collective action.

Innovations in Urban Agriculture

The future of urban food production is being shaped by technological and social innovations:

Vertical Farms: Large-scale vertical farming systems are transforming urban spaces into high-yield food production hubs.

Smart Gardening Tools: Internet of Things (IoT) devices, sensors, and apps make urban gardening more efficient and accessible.

Policy Support: Governments are increasingly recognizing the value of urban agriculture and providing incentives for rooftop gardens, green walls, and urban farms.

Urban gardening is poised to play a pivotal role in creating resilient, sustainable cities that prioritize the well-being of their residents and the planet.

Urban gardening is more than a method of growing food; it is a lifestyle that empowers individuals, strengthens communities, and contributes to a sustainable future. Reflecting on your journey highlights your growth as a gardener and the rewards of your efforts. Expanding your garden opens new possibilities for creativity, productivity, and sustainability.

As urbanization continues, the importance of urban gardening will only grow. It offers a pathway to address pressing global challenges like food insecurity, climate change, and resource scarcity. By embracing this practice, you become part of a movement that not only enriches your life but also transforms cities into greener, more resilient spaces.

The future of urban food production is bright, and your garden—no matter how small—is a vital part of it. Keep growing, experimenting, and sharing your knowledge, for urban gardening is not just about planting seeds in the soil but about sowing the seeds of change for a better

world.

9 798303 922808